Love Your Heart, Love Aerobics

Proven Life Hacks on How to Keep Doing Aerobics

By: Cynthia Lopez

9781681275253

Publishers Notes

Disclaimer – Speedy Publishing LLC

This publication is intended to provide helpful and informative material. It is not intended to diagnose, treat, cure, or prevent any health problem or condition, nor is intended to replace the advice of a physician. No action should be taken solely on the contents of this book. Always consult your physician or qualified health-care professional on any matters regarding your health and before adopting any suggestions in this book or drawing inferences from it.

The author and publisher specifically disclaim all responsibility for any liability, loss or risk, personal or otherwise, which is incurred as a consequence, directly or indirectly, from the use or application of any contents of this book.

Any and all product names referenced within this book are the trademarks of their respective owners. None of these owners have sponsored, authorized, endorsed, or approved this book.

Always read all information provided by the manufacturers' product labels before using their products. The author and publisher are not responsible for claims made by manufacturers.

This book was originally printed before 2014. This is an adapted reprint by Speedy Publishing LLC with newly updated content designed to help readers with much more accurate and timely information and data.

Speedy Publishing LLC

40 E Main Street, Newark, Delaware, 19711

Contact Us: 1-888-248-4521

Website: http://www.speedypublishing.co

REPRINTED Paperback Edition: 9781681275253:

Manufactured in the United States of America

Dedication

This book is dedicated to John. You have done this country great service when you enlisted. Thank you.

TABLE OF CONTENTS

CHAPTER 1- A COMPLETE LIST OF THE BENEFITS OF AEROBICS

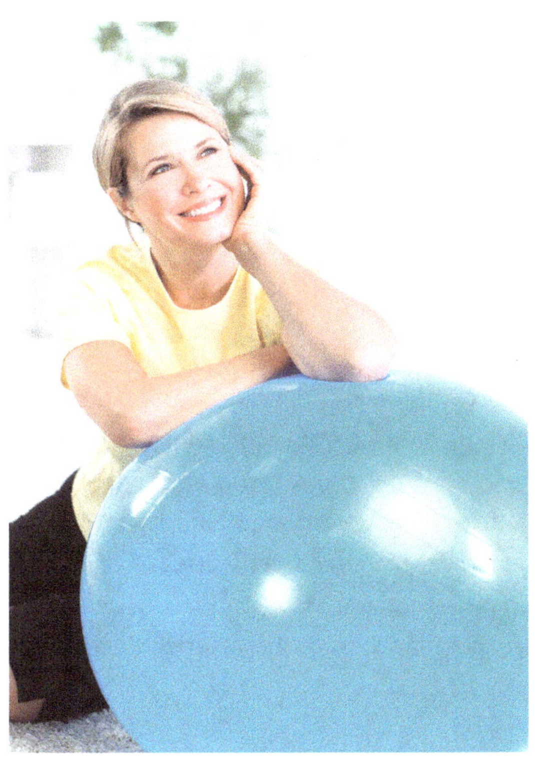

We are always reminded that exercise could do wonders for the body. Aerobics, a kind of exercise which helps your body use more oxygen while maintaining your target heart range; can definitely help a person live longer and healthier. There are studies showing that 30 minutes of aerobics every day would benefit the body a lot.

Performing regular aerobic exercises would gradually make the heart larger. A bigger and larger heart would be able to provide more oxygenated blood which can be used by the muscles. This could also mean more energy whether for longer or shorter periods of exercise or physical activities.

• Weight loss

Aerobics and any kind of physical activity could surely help control and reduce weight. It is most successful when combined with a healthy diet. Including physical activity and exercise with your daily routine will surely help you achieve better built, healthy lifestyle and increase in energy. Aerobics would help your body burn the calories consumed and prevent them from becoming accumulated fats.

• Stronger resistance against sickness

Aerobics can boost the body's immune system. This would prevent illnesses like colds and flu from happening. It could also help the body manage existing health problems like high blood pressure and blood sugar. Excessive weight and obesity could cause serious health problems like diabetes, heart disease and stroke. Aerobics could help in reducing the risks of these diseases. This kind of exercise could help in clearing the arteries of the heart from bad cholesterol.

• Elderly benefits

Aging could have different effects on the body and exercise could help you deal with these changes. It could help your body become stronger and more mobile when you grow old. Common problems of the elderly would be flexibility and mobility. Aerobics and maintaining other forms of exercise even when older would help reduce these problems.

• Increase in stamina and energy

Contrary to what some people think, aerobics and exercise wouldn't leave you breathless and less energetic. It could boost your stamina and energy. Continuous and regular exercise could result to muscle development and increase in body endurance. Aside from that, aerobics could also reduce fatigue and decrease shortness of breath. Aerobics could help the body achieve better sleep at night, making the person more energetic and fresh the next day.

• Promote better mental health

Exercise does not only calm and help the body; it could also help in boosting a mood of a person. Achieving better health and physical results through aerobics could increase self-esteem and self-confidence. It is even used to reduce stress, anxiety and depression.

Aerobics have numerous benefits. In fact, some would say that aside from physical and mental benefits, aerobics could also help in improving sexual performance. There are also different types of aerobic exercises which could capture the interest of people with different ages and characteristics.

However, aerobics may not be safe for everybody. Those with certain illnesses and those that are pregnant should take necessary precautions when performing aerobic exercises. Before trying any aerobic routine, it is important to consult with a doctor first especially if you have an existing or past medical condition.

• Stronger lungs and heart

Doing aerobics help your lung muscles to gain more strength to breathe. If you have any chronic illnesses, such as bronchitis or asthma, aerobics can help with that as well. These illnesses, along with emphysema, will help you to breathe better. Aerobics also helps you to gain an advantage with oxygen for your lungs.

Love Your Heart, Love Aerobics
If you do aerobics at least three times every week, your heart rate will increase. Your heart will also be able to pump additional blood into your body. Your muscles will get oxygen at a quicker rate.

- **Toner muscles**

Your muscles will gain more strength when you do aerobics. They also get larger and your body will become leaner because you will have more muscle mass. Your muscles will also increase in body fat so that you will have more energy. Your metabolism will increase due to the lean muscle, which results in you losing more weight.

CHAPTER 2- DO AEROBICS EVERYWHERE

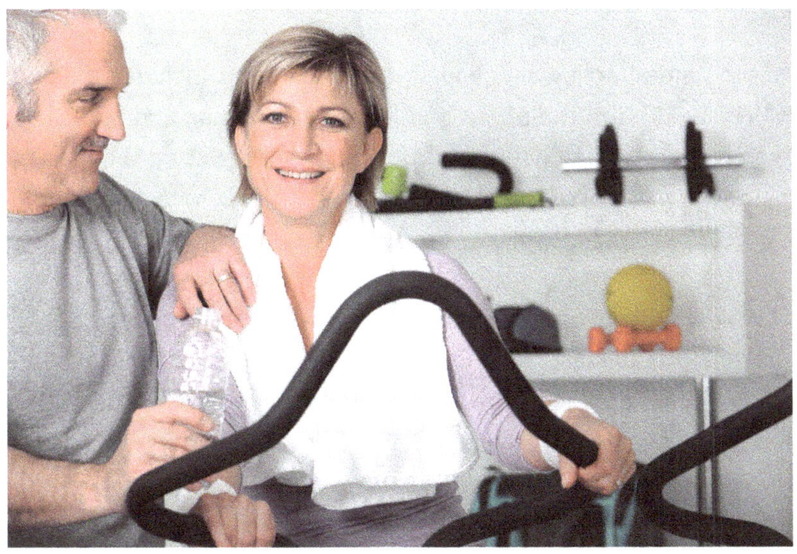

Aerobics is one of the most popular types of exercises in the market. Its use of music, dance, equipment and other facilities have contributed to its popularity. Aerobic exercises are workouts that intend to increase the heart rate for a period of time. This would cause the body to have higher intake of oxygen which would result into better blood circulation, weight loss, faster calorie and fat burning.

Other physical activities can also be considered as aerobic workouts, like swimming, running, walking, jogging, and cycling. An aerobic exercise would start with a 5 to 10 minutes of warm-up stretching and exercises. After the warming-up, the routine proper would follow, lasting for about 20 to 30 minutes. The last part of the workout will be the cooling-down process.

There are different types of aerobic exercises for different levels of individuals. Skill, health and comfort are things to be considered when choosing what type of aerobic exercise would fit with the individual's needs and abilities. Some of the types are:

• Low-impact aerobics

As the name implies, low-impact exercises don't include activities which could harm the bones and joints like jumping and bouncing. Exercises performed had lower intensity, thus reducing the risks of injuries and leg overuse. In this exercise, one or both feet should always be in contact with the ground.

With low-impact routine, you do not start with a high note. An individual could start performing the exercises on a slower rate and gradually increase its intensity. Low-impact aerobics is ideal for seniors, obese and overweight individuals and of course, pregnant women.

• High impact aerobics

High impact aerobic exercises use different movements. It could include jumping, turning, shuffling, doubling, etc. This kind of workout intends to develop the abdominal area, calf, and also the cardiovascular system. If an individual is agile and active prior to working out, then high-impact aerobics may be the best option. But for beginners, slower and low-impact exercises is recommended first. When the individual is already comfortable with this low-impact level, then it would be safe to proceed with the second level. Keep in mind that doctor's discretion is always important.

• Step Aerobics

Step aerobics uses step benches for working out. This kind of aerobics is actually low in impact. There are studies showing that step aerobics can help a person reduce weight, given the fact that its impact is only half of the impact used when riding a bike at home. Overall, this process or workout is dedicated for the development of the lower body.

• Aerobic kickboxing

It is also called cardio boxing. This is one of the most effective workouts for losing weight. Although, aerobic kickboxing is tiring, its effects on the body are great. It could definitely help in building more energy and longer stamina. It is also called cardio boxing and can burn about 800 calories in an hour.

• Water aerobics

Another low-impact exercise but delivers huge results, whether it is for weight loss or improving over-all health. Water aerobics, according to experts, burns calories faster compared with land-exercises because of the water's resistance.

Can You Do Aerobics from Home?

If taking an aerobics class is out of your budget, then you can do them at home. In fact, it's probably easier to do because you can be more relaxed and you don't have to use gas to go anywhere. The exercises can be done in the comfort of your own home. It does not matter how you look because no one will see you.

Aerobic is an easy exercise routine to start out at home. If you are one of those people who have not worked out in a while and your body is not looking its best, doing aerobics at home can help you from being embarrassed in front of others. Once you get into shape, you can venture outside to take some classes.

Love Your Heart, Love Aerobics
Just because you are doing aerobics at home does not mean that you won't get the same benefits that you would if you were in a class. You would still be able to enhance your health and get your heart and lungs strong, lose weight and be able to reduce stress.

Even though you are at home, you should do aerobics exercises starting at three times a week, 30 minutes a day and work your way up. You can increase the intensity of your sessions as you feel you are ready.

You can use a treadmill to work out. You can probably one that is one sale. Treadmills don't cost a lot either.

You can also use aerobic exercise videos to get you started. You may have to watch it once or twice to get the hang of what's going on. There is step aerobics, dancing, kickboxing and other different styles of aerobics. Start out at the level that you feel most comfortable with. For many people, that would be the beginning level.

Videos can be bought from retailers such as Wal-Mart or Target. Or if you don't want to go out, you can order them online. They videos usually come in a series, so you would get the benefit of doing several different aerobic exercises.

If you feel that you are not disciplined enough to do this on your own, then you must find a partner. It could be your spouse, a friend or your children, provided that they are old enough.

Having a partner can help you with that support that you need to keep going when you want to quit. Even if you're not thinking about quitting, a partner can help you to the next level.

Try and do your aerobic exercises when there are no other people around. That way you won't be interrupted.

How to Warm-Up Properly

There's no doubt—you must warm up before you start running. Make it a habit every time you run to warm up. It is an important part of your aerobic exercise. You can prevent unnecessary injuries. Many sports athletes know that they have to do this before every game or else they can risk being injured. You are no different in that aspect. Your muscles need to be loose before you start moving.

You can warm up your muscles for about 10 – 15 minutes and make them flexible. If your muscles are cold and you don't warm them up, you will not get the output that you desire. You could also pull a muscle in the process.

You can do light cardiovascular exercises in order for the blood to flow through your body. Light jogging is another way that you can warm up before you start running. Whatever you use for warm up exercises, they should be low impact and light, such as lunges.

Don't rest after you have warmed up. Do some stretching so that you will keep your momentum going. You want to be ready to run right after you're finished. Don't overstretch your joints and muscles or you could cause injury to those areas.

Then you can start running and get into your exercise.

CHAPTER 3- STEPPING UP WEIGHT LOSS WITH THE STEP AEROBICS

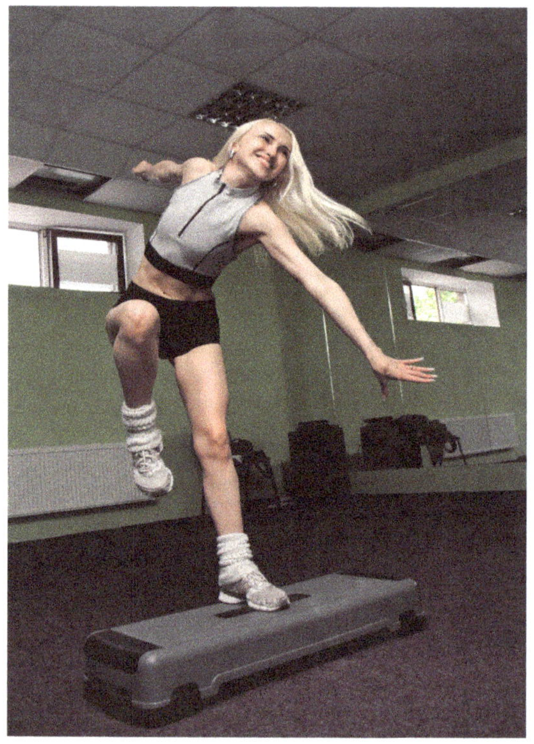

This style of aerobics uses a platform that is elevated. This aerobics is very popular with a lot of people. You will exercise with music that has a fast beat along with steps that coordinate with the beats. You will find this kind of aerobics exercise performed at health clubs and gyms as a class. However, you can purchase a step aerobics package and do it on your own at home.

The platform raises no more than a foot off the ground. The sessions are usually no longer than an hour. However, there are some half-hour sessions as well. How it works is you will step on and off of the platform according to the beat of the music. There are different ways of stepping where you have to use the platform.

You can burn calories using step aerobics. Your muscles will also get strong and your metabolism will increase. The oxygen in your body will increase. Your heart will beat faster and build up stamina. Once your heart gets up to speed, more blood will be able to flow to your body.

This is a low impact exercise. You have to make sure that you are doing it right, otherwise you could hurt your knees and joints. Whether you are following a video or an instructor, you must pay attention to every step. You should be wearing shoes that are comfortable and made to perform exercises of this kind. They should have rubber on the bottom that is not slippery.

If you have never done step aerobics before, please consult with your physician prior to starting.

Getting Ready for Step Aerobics

Using these precautions before you start your step aerobics workout will help you to get the best out of it. It will also help prevent injuries that can be inflicted if you don't do it correctly.

Before you start, make sure that you are in good enough shape to start this aerobic exercise. Otherwise, you will find yourself out of breath before you get into it good enough.

Your foot should be on the step. It should be the entire foot, not part of it. You need to be able to balance well when you are stepping on and off. If you don't you could lose your balance and possibly fall or injure yourself. This is crucial if you are stepping to fast music.

The knees should measure up over your ankles. Don't do lunges as you are stepping up on to the platform. You want to make sure that the knee stays over the ankle each time you step up.

Only use so many risers with the step. Two or three risers should be the recommended amount, depending on your height. The stepper needs to be comfortable enough where you won't endure stress with your back and your knees.

Keep a straight posture as you step up and down. Do not bend your back or hips forward. When you are doing step aerobics, skip the hand or ankle weights. Using weights while you are stepping can cause injuries to your knees, shoulders and ankles. You are already moving fast and having weights is an extra burden that can stress out the joints.

Chapter 4- Having Fun while Wading in Water Aerobics

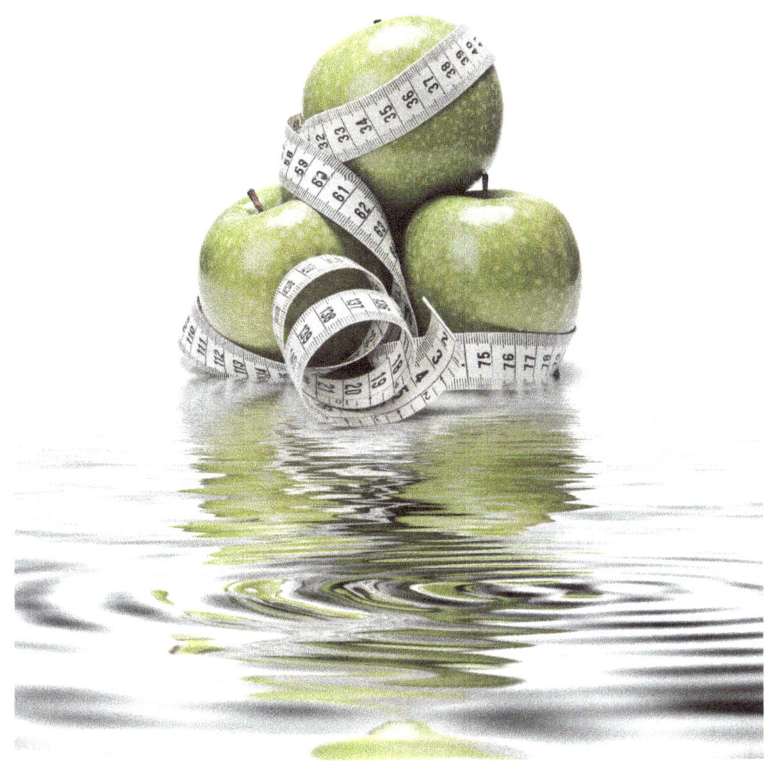

Physical activities like walking, running, dancing and swimming can be considered aerobics. Aerobics are exercises which increase the heart rate and at the same time pump more oxygen into the blood vessels. There are different kinds of aerobic exercises which can be defined based on the equipment used in the workout program. Water aerobic workout is an example of an aerobic workout.

Water aerobics or aqua aerobics can also be referred to as waterobics. This kind of workout is usually performed in a swimming pool with waist-deep water. It could be in an indoor or outdoor pool, with water temperature of 82º F to 86º F. Come to think of it, the most common form of waterobics is swimming.

Love Your Heart, Love Aerobics
Water aerobics would focus on building body strength, flexibility, balance and providing a cardiovascular workout. One session usually lasts for about 40 to 50 minutes.

Just like any other aerobic workout, there is a five-minute warm-up and would end with five-minute cool-down. There could be floatation devices provided to the participants if the water is deep. Kickboards and water barbells are also provided to help participants afloat or can be used for exercises. Water weights and floating belts are also used to increase water resistance. Music is used during workout sessions.

When kicking off with waterobics, the most basic thing that you need is your swimsuit. There are some participants who would also use a swimming cap to keep the hair out of the face and special aqua shoes. These special shoes can support you ankles and also prevent your feet from slipping. They would also serve as protection against cuts and scrapes.

There are numerous benefits from including water aerobics in your lifestyle.

• Since water provides buoyancy and support to the body, there are fewer risks of bone and joint injury, which makes it ideal for seniors who are suffering from arthritis or back pains. Working out in water makes an individual less achy and sore after the workout. Body joints did not have any problem with maximizing its movement.

• Some would say that they experienced faster shaping and toning of muscles when doing water exercises, compared with conducting them on land. Water aerobics could help the muscles develop 12 to 14 times faster than it does when doing in land. Since water has higher density than air, it has higher resistance which is among the reasons for better muscular development and endurance

- The heart works better when doing water aerobics. Compared to activities like running or swimming, the heart rate is maintained at a lower rate.

- This is great for burning calories and losing weight. Walking for instance, when done on land can burn about 135 calories in half an hour. If performed in water, you could burn by as much as 264 calories for the 30-minute session.

- Aqua aerobics are great for those who have arthritis, osteoporosis and pregnant because the workouts are actually gentle enough for joint movements but quick enough to build muscle mass. Still, if a person has the following medical conditions, expert's advice is still important.

Even with all the benefits, water aerobics is still not perfect. Since it would require the use of facilities and equipment, water aerobics exercise tend to be more expensive. Some health insurance providers could provide coverage for the aqua aerobics as long as it is recommended by the attending physician.

Chapter 5- Breathing, Dancing and Other Aerobic Essentials

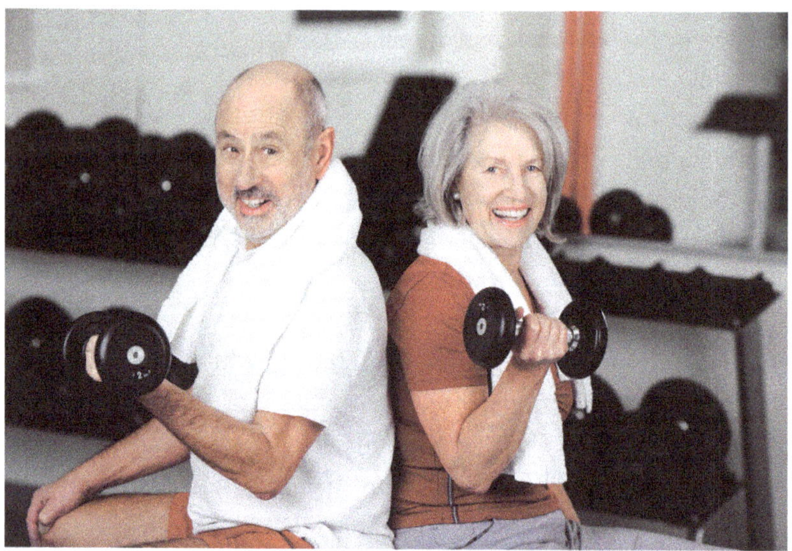

• Breathing

Aerobics is one of the ways to lose weight and reduce risks of sickness and complications as a result of obesity and being overweight. It will also improve overall health. Aerobics could help in pumping more oxygen into the blood vessels, which can increase metabolism and burn more fat and calories. Aerobics literally means oxygen. Aerobic exercises are designed to increase oxygen intake. This practice would burn fat and improve health and fitness.

According to studies, about 300,000 adult deaths in the United States can be attributed to the lack of physical activity and unhealthy eating habits. About two thirds of adults in the U.S. are overweight, while about one-third of the adult population is obese. Adults are not the only ones suffering from weight problems. Children and teens with obesity have increased for the last years because of changes in lifestyle.

Cynthia Lopez
Would it be possible then to lose weight just by breathing alone?

Breathing is a crucial aspect in different kinds of exercises. In fact, in yoga, breathing properly is important. Breathing exercises could even remove stress and relax the body and mind. Breathing for weight loss is practiced by several aerobic breathing programs. Each program would have its own technique and advice.

However, it is important to understand that there is no weight loss program or pill that could produce dramatic results overnight. Obesity and being overweight cannot be resolved by aerobic breathing alone. Of course, proper diet and exercise is still crucial to battle the pounds away. Aerobic breathing can supplement these weight loss programs to acquire better results.

Most of us would only use about 20% of our lung capacity, while 70% of toxic elimination in our body happens when we breathe. Aerobic breathing helps our body maximize its potential. By breathing properly for about 20 minutes a day, you can bring drastic results in your health.

The guiding principle is that breathing can cleanse your body. It could help in flushing out waste, toxins and other pollutants from your body. Diaphragmatic deep breathing techniques could help in reducing cellulite; improve skin tone, blood circulation, digestion and even sleep.

With aerobic breathing, all you have to do is sit up straight, exhale from the lungs and inhale through the nose. Breathing should be able to stretch the lungs to its capacity. When exhaling, make sure to force out all the air in the lungs. Hold breathing for a while and then pull your stomach in. You can do these breathing exercises about 10 to 20 times. Some would prefer doing them before proceeding with any exercise training.

Everyone wants to lose weight. But it does not mean that you should start starving yourself and become a slave to exercise machines. In the end, losing weight would still mean eating fruits, vegetables and healthy food, exercising regularly and staying or maintaining a positive outlook of life.

Whenever we are including ourselves in aerobics and weight loss programs, setting realistic goals for us to accomplish would make it easier for us and at the same time, take weight loss according to our own phase. Breathing may not be the magic beans we're looking for to look good, but it can definitely help us change into a new person.

• Dancing

Aerobic dancing combines exercises and different forms of dances like ballet and jazz into an exercise routine. They are usually considered low-impact exercises and slower paced compared with other aerobic routines, although there are also fast-paced routines. Because of these characteristics, they are very ideal for those who need low-impact routines like the elderly, overweight and those who are pregnant.

What makes aerobic dance an interesting routine is, of course, its music. There are different types of music which can be used for different aerobic dances; there are different speed and style variations of aerobic dances. There are guidelines for aerobic music. It is usually about 120 to 124 beats per minute for step aerobics. For low-impact exercises, it is usually about 136 to 148 beats per minute. Beginners would dance or sweat it out with slower beats.

Aerobic dance could be classified into high-impact exercises, low-impact, step aerobics and water dance aerobics. High impact exercises, as its name implies, would involve intensive exercises which includes jumping actions synchronized with the music. Step aerobics uses the step bench, and the water aerobics is performed in waist-deep water.

Aside from the movements along with the music, aerobic dance is also combined with fast or aerobic breathing. This pumps more oxygen into the blood stream, rejuvenating the body. Aerobic dances are usually done from 20 to 30 minutes, practiced for three times a week. The routine is performed just like rhythmic dances, with counts essential in setting the rhythm.

Before proceeding with the routine, getting warmed-up is important. It would usually last for 10 to 15 minutes. These stretching exercises will lower risks of injury and at the same time prepare the body for any extensive movement. After the routine proper, relaxing or cooling down movements for another 5 to 15 minutes will be performed to help the heart and the muscles relax.

Aerobic dancing has many benefits even though they were done or practiced in a fun way. This kind of aerobic workout is a great way to lose weight and at the same time, tone body muscles. It would also help the body develop strength among bones who carry most the body's weight and also toughen cardiovascular muscles.

Just like other exercises, aerobic dance can increase the circulation of the blood; reduce the levels of blood sugar and cholesterol. Because aerobic dancing would include proper breathing exercises, more oxygen is circulated in the heart, lungs and blood vessels which makes the body to function better, produce higher energy and stamina. Its physical benefits would also include boosting of the immune system, preparing the body against colds, flu, etc.

Aerobic dancing is also a great way to keep stress away. This could break the stressful and monotonous routine we have at home, school or in the work place. It can even allow you to develop or practice your creativity, since you can create your own dance steps or routine. If you cannot leave the house to go to a gym, you could do the aerobic exercises at home, learn the steps and pick your own song. How fun it is to stay healthy with aerobics by swaying your hips!

• Needed Aerobic Equipment

Aerobics is not only good for your body but also for your overall health. It is also a great way of losing weight and keeping the unwanted pounds away. Although aerobic exercises are good as it is like kickboxing, walking, jogging or similar routines, using aerobic equipment would make exercising more fun and at the same time burn calories faster.

There are different kinds of equipment which could be used for different aerobic exercises.

• Step bench

This is the most common equipment. The height of the step depends on the leg movements that would be used. Of course, the height would depend on the experience and expertise of the person using it. Usually, a beginner would start with a 4-inch step. As the person becomes more experienced, the height would increase to build more endurance and flexibility. One thing great about aerobic steps is that it is portable enough to be carried anywhere.

When buying a step bench, a bench with a non-slip surface will be a good idea since it would more safe. Just keep in mind that a higher step bench would mean a more intense workout.

• Stationary Bicycle

Unlike ordinary bicycles there are located only in one place. To measure the progress of the bike, an ergometer is installed. There are even stationary bikes which have computers that contain the exercise data and sessions. These bikes have different features which influence the costs of the equipment. There are different kinds of stationary bikes; buying one does not mean you would have to pick the most sophisticated and expensive model. The needs of the user come first.

• Treadmill

Treadmills can be expensive. There are manual and motorized treadmills which can be bought from different fitness centers. There are different features included in a treadmill like the pulse monitor, bottle holder, and book rack. There are even sophisticated models which would allow you to use video and audio players to kill boredom while doing the exercises. When buying treadmill, the size is the most important factor. Check if it would be able to fit into your exercise or living room area.

• Hand weights

Lifting weights is another component of aerobic exercises. When seriously trying to build muscles, then start getting 3 lbs. and 5 lbs. weights. When using hand weights, users are recommended to use aerobic gloves to grip better. Water aerobics also have customized weights which can be used in aquatic exercises.

Love Your Heart, Love Aerobics

Whenever performing aerobic exercises, using the proper gear is important, the right clothes and shoes. Make sure that the clothes will allow the body to move easily, the shoes should be comfortable enough and keep the user balanced.

Aside from paying attention to wearing the proper working-out clothes, asking your doctor or health-care provider about any kind of recommendation with what kind of fitness equipment and program would be suitable for your needs is important. If buying fitness equipment is out of the option, then you could always sign-up for a membership in fitness centers, as long as they offer the equipment you would prefer to use.

CHAPTER 6 - LOSE CALORIES THROUGH AEROBIC KICKBOXING

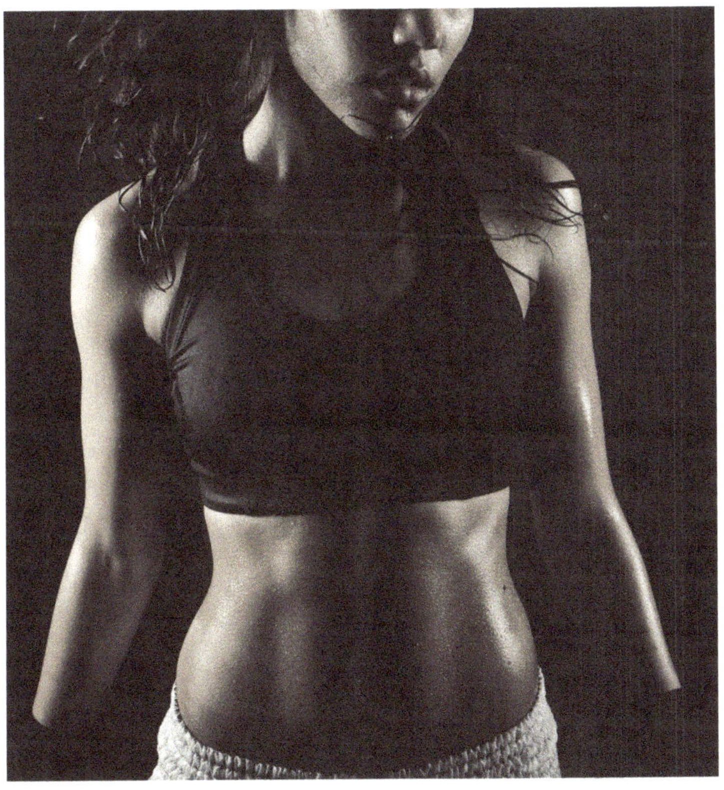

There are different types and routines in aerobics. And one of them is aerobic kickboxing. Aerobic kickboxing should not be confused with kickboxing which is a self-defense technique. With aerobic kickboxing, which is also called cardio kickboxing, you could lose about 800 calories within an hour. Aside from losing weight, cardio kickboxing is also great in building lower and upper body strength.

Aerobic kickboxing starts just like any other kind of aerobic exercise, with five to ten minutes of warm-up. After that, it would be the kicking and punching which would end up with another five minute cool-down. This aerobic exercise combines martial-arts, self-defense, boxing and music. A person who is performing this would be able to learn the basics of these parts. For example, basic boxing stance is taught. Punches like jabs and hooks, kicks like sidekicks are taught.

Kickboxing is thought to have originated from Muay Thai. But aside from the Thai boxing influences, aerobic kickboxing also uses karate skills to develop flexibility, strength and endurance in one cardiovascular exercise. Those who practice aerobic kickboxing would also testify that it was able to help them build their self-confidence, self-esteem, self-control and develop a positive attitude towards exercising and work-out.

In addition to that, it can also reduce levels of stress and increase the individual's stamina and energy. Imagine, learning self-defense and keeping your personal fitness in check in an hour or less in a day. But as great as it is, there should be considerations before practicing aerobic kickboxing.

• Your personal level of fitness.

Aerobic kickboxing is a high-impact aerobic routine. Those who are suffering from arthritis, tight hamstrings and inflexible back can have difficulties with this routine. And always consider getting your doctor's advice before proceeding with any kind of exercise program especially if you have an existing medical condition.

• Consider your level of expertise.

If it is your first time to do such workout, then you could always get a beginning class. After being familiar with it, you could start progressing into intermediate and advance levels. If working out with a CD/DVD or tape at home, then pay attention to the instructions and start and do the workout according to your own pace. There are moves like high-kicks which should be avoided by beginners. These moves would require flexibility which would be developed later on when you have already gotten used to the routine.

• Hydrate.

Always drink water before, during and after the workout.

• If the CD or the class runs for more than an hour, you are not obligated to work out for the entire period. An hour of aerobic exercise is enough.

• Wear clothes that would not restrict the flow of movements while exercising. Loose-fitting clothes could be a problem sometimes.

Cardio kickboxing could still put beginners at risk of joint injury. Especially, if they would be extending or using incorrect forms and stances like overextending kicks and locking joints. Wearing weights and holding dumbbells are also not a good idea since they could also be detrimental to your joints. When performing aerobic kickboxing or any kind of aerobics, never give in to peer pressure and excise beyond your limits or fatigue.

Keep in mind that speed, flexibility and your overall performance and fitness will increase along with regular practice.

Chapter 7- Can Children and Pregnant Women do Aerobics Too?

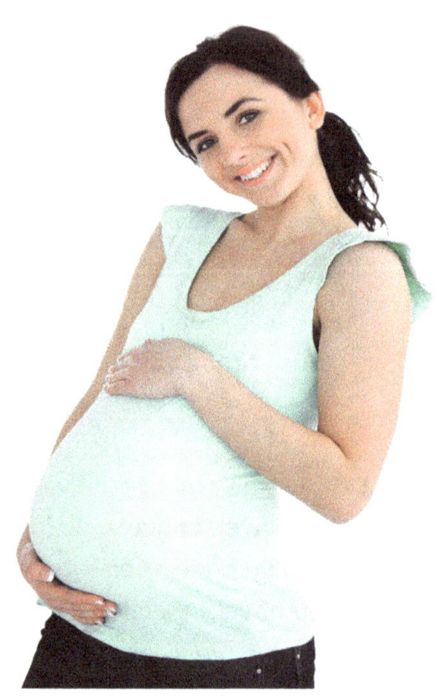

It is important to teach kids early about health and fitness. Involving them in exercise and aerobics would not only help them understand health but also help them direct their energies into movements and practices that would be productive and at the same time, beneficial in the long run.

According to studies, about 25% of children and teens do not have any "vigorous physical activity." About 14% children and teens report no physical activity like walking or cycling, every day. This can be one of the reasons why the number of children has doubled since the early 1970s. In 2000, 19% of children, 6 to 11 years old, and 17%, 12 to 19 years old, are considered overweight.

Cynthia Lopez

Those who are involved in physical activities, reduce the risks of developing health problems as they grow older. Exercising reduces the risks of obesity, diabetes, high blood pressure, stroke and heart disease. But making your child follow a 30 minute exercise video is no fun for your kid. There are fitness centers that have children workout program, they would include biking, swimming, walking, marching, playing games to introduce low, moderate and high impact aerobics and physical activity.

Introducing children and teens to aerobics would help them become more active and at the same time, change their outlook towards the lifestyle they will be having as they grow old. There are also fitness centers which offer exercise programs suitable for children and teens, based on their age, skill and of course, their fitness and personal condition.

There are also CDs and DVDs that mix an aerobic workout with dances and other fun ways. Teens and older children may enjoy dancing to hip-hop and modern dances. Some would also show interest in doing aerobics dances, kickboxing, yoga and Pilates. You could also help your child participate in school-organized sports and activities.

There are guidelines that should be kept in mind when involving your child in physical activity according to Centers for Disease Control and Prevention (1997) and the Council for Physical Education for Children (1998). Children should at least be physically active within 30 to 60 minutes on all or most of the days of the week. Moderate to vigorous activity a day should last for about 10 to 15 minutes. Playing games and activities like biking, walking, running, etc. should also be included in the child's activities.

To encourage physical activity, make sure to implement rules that would lead to healthier lifestyle. This would include setting time for watching television and computer games. Aside from that, make sure that your child would be eating meals not in front of the television or computer. This would promote or give time for parents to talk to children during meals.

The easiest way to teach and encourage children to exercise is to set an example. Obesity and overweight problems are not just children health concerns, alarmingly, a lot of adults also suffer from these health problems. The family exercising together helps the family build stronger and closer relationships. Aerobics would not only benefit your child, but the whole family as well.

Careful Exercises for Pregnancy

Everybody can benefit from exercise, even those who are handicapped. The elderly would exhibit health improvements when performing low-impact exercises. Pregnant women would also benefit from low-impact aerobic exercises. Those who practice aerobics while pregnant would experience easier labor and child-birth.

There are also studies that showed women who have been performing aerobic exercises have reduced risk of undergoing caesarean operation/ surgery, quicker recovery whether it is physical or from postpartum depression. These women would also shed pounds gained during pregnancy, faster. Overall, women would testify that they had healthier pregnancy compared with other women.

Exercising while pregnant does not mean that soon-to-be-mothers would carry on the same pace or exercises they were doing prior to pregnancy. Since expecting mothers are practically sustaining two lives in their bodies, they should not be exerting too much in their exercises. Pregnant women are recommended to perform aerobic exercises for not more than 30 minutes. When exercising too much, the body temperature of both mother and child could increase. This could cause problems with the baby; excessive heat during the first trimester could cause birth defects. While later on during second trimester, it could trigger premature birth.

To avoid hyperthermia or excessive heat, exercises can be performed early in the morning when the weather is cooler. Pregnant women should drink plenty of water and avoid exerting too much force or energy, like weightlifting. Places like saunas and steam rooms should be avoided. As all pregnant women know, exercises which would make the abdomen and the stomach vulnerable should be avoided by all means. Jumping movements should also be avoided.

Light weight-lifting can also be practiced by pregnant women. This would be able to prepare them for carrying the baby after birth. Although, experts would always recommend that before proceeding to any kind of aerobic routine or program, doctor's advice is very important. Other forms of exercise which could be carried out during the first trimester would include swimming, walking, and there are special aerobic programs designed for pregnant women. While exercising, it is important to keep eat and keep your body hydrated.

During the second and last trimester, the weight of the baby could have an effect on your movements. Maintaining your balance is hard since the weight could provide stress in your joints. During this time, marching in place could replace your usual exercise routine. Exercises which would require you to bend over, spin and quick turning movements can cause the mother to lose balance and result into injury.

Love Your Heart, Love Aerobics

Use caution as you move across the floor. You may want to try a prenatal water aerobics class if one is offered in your community. It offers many of the same benefits as aerobics on land- a workout for your heart and body and the camaraderie of other expectant mothers without the stress on your joints or the risk of injury or a fall.

Even though aerobics has many benefits, doctors may not recommend it to some pregnant moms especially if they show signs of preeclampsia or worsening hypertension. The American College of Obstetricians and Gynecologists (ACOG) also cautions pregnant women against aerobic exercises that would require them to lie on their backs when they're about 20 weeks pregnant. Generally, if a pregnant woman is experiencing unusual symptoms like pain, bleeding, rapid heartbeat or dizziness, exercises should be stopped.

Chapter 8- Aerobics and Weight Loss

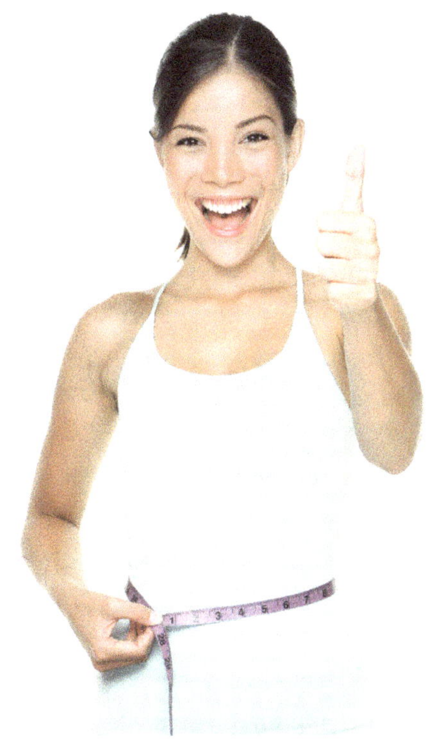

One of the most popular means of losing weight ever since is aerobic exercises because of its long term benefits when it comes to overall health. Although many people are living testaments to the wonders of weight loss by dieting and cutting down on important nutrients, not all of these offer certain and desirable results like aerobic exercises can.

If you are one of those who are contemplating over losing weight, then now is the time to stop entertaining the thoughts on weight loss programs or diets. It is now time to conduct a little research first on aerobic exercises to help you understand how aerobics help you lose weight and achieve can long term health benefits.

Basics of Aerobics

Aerobics refer to doing an activity such as a physical exercise for a longer period of time but with lesser force and effort on the part of the one who is doing it. Simply put aerobics exercises are those that allow a person to do multi-tasking such as carrying out a conversation while doing the exercise or engaging in simple yet productive activities.

The most common forms of aerobic exercises might include simple walking, jogging, swimming and even cross country skiing. To those who cannot carry on these simple exercises religiously on their own, they can try attending aerobic classes nearby where there is an instructor to lead them.

Experts say that before you engage in any activity such as aerobic exercises please make sure that you have reviewed its requirements well. Avoid choosing activities that would not suit your health and lifestyle conditions.

Also, make sure that you have visited a registered or licensed physician first before trying on aerobic exercises and before using any weight loss product that you think might complement your activity such as food supplements, herbs, or over-the-counter medications.

What Can You Do?

To ensure that aerobic exercises will work for you, take time off to read and understand various issues surrounding it. You can check the Internet where there are thousands of sites that will lead you into any information you want on aerobic exercise or ask a person who you know that did this before so you can ask for first hand tips and suggestions. It will also help if you:

- record your eating habits and patterns by keeping a food journal. Updating and monitoring your food and eating patterns will help you track down the reasons behind your weight gain. Asking for professional help from a registered dietitian will make the monitoring more valid.

- indulge and give in if you are craving for a specific food or dish since being not overly-restrictive with food or favorite treats can be awarding experience. By giving into these cravings you can totally avoid eating foods that are high in calories and fats.

- engage yourself in only one daily exercise such as walking—which is the easiest form of aerobic exercise—since it is recommended by most authorities to help you lose weight while keeping your body fit and healthy. Other exercises and workouts that last 30 to 60 minutes will also help you burn unwanted fats and calories.

Today, more and more remedies are being offered in the market for those people who would want to lose weight. Among these are weight loss remedies come in the form of products, supplements, and programs. But if there is one thing that experts would consider the safest, it would be aerobic exercises.

Before you engage in any weight loss diet, product, or program, make sure that you have full comprehension of its effects and possible side effects to avoid going back to your form after you lose weight. Being knowledgeable about these products and the possible risks associated with it can give you an idea what are the products you can take in, diets you can engage in or programs you can enroll with.

Most studies show that diets that promote weight loss of more than two pounds weekly are not safe because it increases the possibility of serious health problems compared to gradual weight loss. Medical experts also agree that losing weight at a slower rate may reduce risks of health problems that are closely associated with rapid weight loss.

Also, fad diets and quick weight loss products available today do not only ignore but totally violates the basic principles of good nutrition and various dietary guidelines. Do not be overwhelmed with the promise of quick weight loss because any claims that a person can lose weight almost effortlessly are fabricated.

These are just some of the reasons why more and more experts recommend safe means of cutting down on weight such as aerobics. Since aerobic exercises entail doing a lesser effort in an activity for a longer period of time, many say that this could be an effective tool to achieve long term health benefits.

How to Keep Doing Aerobic Exercises

Aside serious health risks and psychological impacts brought by futile dieting, improper weight loss through the use of non-prescribed weight loss products or diets that are not proven to be effective can bring depression plus a weakened immune system. This is why experts strongly recommend safe means of being fit and slim through aerobic exercises.

Many say that losing weight can be frustrating but a rewarding feat once you have achieved your ideal weight and figure. To help you keep up the weight that you have lost in simple aerobic exercises, here are some things that you need to debunk:

- "Low Carb Diet" is the only way for you to lose weight. This is probably one of the biggest lies being promoted by the people of weight loss industry today since by cutting out all carbo and starches will only result to lack of nutrition needed by the body especially by the muscle tissues; and

- A lot of time is needed to work a weight loss program into your schedule. If you think that you cannot handle your weight loss all by yourself, then opt enrolling in a safe and responsible weight loss option such as aerobic classes that can fit into your schedule then you can even do other things for yourself.

Chapter 9 - The Best Aerobic Exercises for All Ages

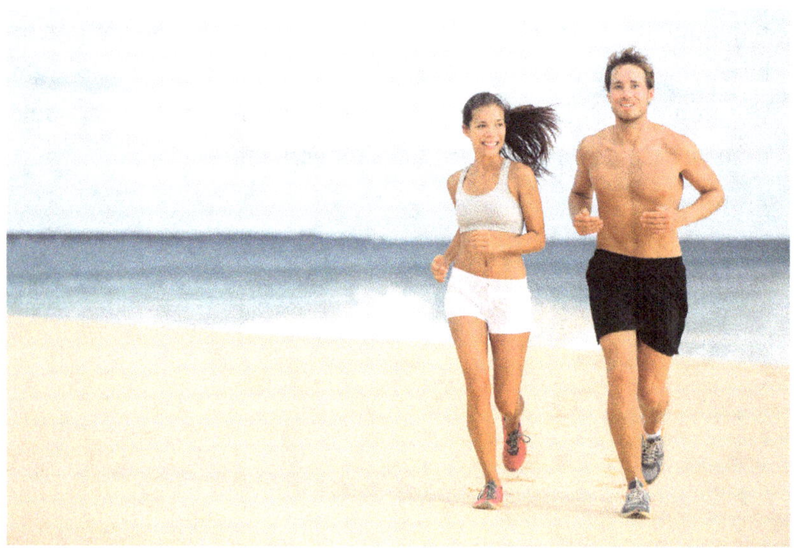

1.Running

Running is one of the best and cost effective ways to get fit. This aerobic exercise can benefit young and old people. When you run, you are doing so at a measured pace. It's faster than a jog, but slower than a complete run. You should run in moderation and don't look to do a hard run. A hard run is not considered aerobic exercising.

Depending on how you function during the day, you can choose to run in the morning or in the afternoons or evening. Everyone does not respond the same when it comes to running.

Before you start, you would have to check out the weather and the environment you would be doing this in. All places are different and there may be some that are not conducive for running. So check out the area before you decide to commit.

You have to prepare yourself for the weather at hand. If it's cool, you will need clothing that will keep your warm. It it's warm, you will need clothing that will keep you cool. You will also need the right kind of shoes to wear when you start running. You will need to be comfortable so that you can get the best fitness workout.

Where Should You Run?

There are different places where you can go running. You can do it in your neighborhood, on a park trail, or anywhere that you feel safe doing this. Make sure that you are running on flat ground or a flat surface.

Don't take the chance running on slopes that are difficult, rough areas or slippery areas. There's a greater chance that you would get injured. The last thing that you need is a sprained ankle or a pulled muscle.

If you are more experienced, there are some slopes and inclines that are made for running. Check out the areas first before you commit to running. Stay near areas where you can get immediate help if needed.

The area where you will be running should not have any obstacles. You need to be free to run so that you can stay on course.

If you find areas where you can run, but they are far away from where you live, find alternative places that are closer and just as good. There may be times when you will not be able to go to those far away spots when you want to.

It's not a bad idea to have a running buddy run with you. They can give you great support.

Always try to go to an area where there are not a lot of other runners. This can throw off your exercise regimen and make you not want to run.

Running Tips

As you run, try to avoid bouncing. If you move up and down too much, you have used up energy that you did not need to use. The lower portion of your body can be affected by this movement. The higher up you are the more shock that is sucked in as you land on the ground. This results in you and your legs getting tired faster than they need to be.

In order to cut the bouncing down to a bare minimum, do some light running and when you land, land on your feet softly. Your feet should be low to the ground level and using brief strides. Your arms should still be at a 90 degree angle and bent. When you swing them, the swing should be shorter and lower.

Don't run on your toes. Running on your toes can contribute to bouncing.

Monitor Your Progress

In order to keep up with your progress, have a log where you can write down the information. Keeping up with this log will help you to see where you are and where you could be. It can be considered as a motivational tool to keep you going. Make sure to keep up with all dates, times and miles. Also, write some comments about that day's exercise.

Don't Rush into Running Fast

When you start running, don't try to be like the NASCAR drivers and take off running. Start off slow and work your way up. Starting out fast does nothing for you accept giving you exhaustion and soreness that you don't need. When you do too much in the beginning, you can also incur unnecessary injuries. Do everything gradually and you will get to your destination. Running will be more fun to you if you don't get ahead of yourself, ending up with stresses and injuries.

Check the Weather

If you are used to running whether it's hot or cold, make sure that you are properly dressed. Having the right clothing makes a difference when you are exercising. You need to feel comfortable while you are running. If the weather is so rough, then find an inside gym where they have running facilities.

Running for Fun

Even though you are running to get fit, don't make it as though it's such a dreadful chore. You want to have fun and be able to release some steam from people or events that rattled you. You also want to improve your health. If you are running outdoors, take in some of the scenery that you would otherwise not get to see.

2. Walking

Walking is one of the easiest aerobics that you can do. Not only does it not cost you anything, but to get up and go, anyone can do it. Whether the pace is slow or fast, walking is good for everyone.

Love Your Heart, Love Aerobics

It only takes 30 minutes a day to complete an effective walking workout. You can start walking three days a week and produce some results. Once you get accustomed to walking, it will be time to do it with more intensity.

Aerobic walking helps to increase your heart and breathing rate. When you start walking every day, you will start to get more fit. You will also be able to avoid some health risks such as cancer, heart ailments and diabetes.

Other benefits of aerobic walking include:

• Having control of your weight

• Muscular fitness

• Being able to balance your body

• Lowers blood pressure

• Less chance of having a stroke or other kinds of cancer

Being injured by walking is not common. It is one of the safest, if not the safest aerobic exercise that everyone can do.

It is recommended that you do at least two and a half hours of aerobic activity every week. That means you can do aerobic walking for 30 minutes a day, five days a week. Even though it may not start out that way, you will eventually work your way up to that point.

Start out by determining how many times a week you will do the aerobic walking. You will need to know how long you will do it for each day that you go out. If you are rusty and have not walked in a while, take your time when you start out.

Some people may do exercises in 10 minute intervals, which is a great idea for the ones who haven't been exercising in a while. Gradually, you will add more time and intensity to your walk. The key is to start out gradually and don't rush to get to the next level.

Before you start, see your physician to get approval for doing this. Not having walked in a while may cause some issues if you don't know what you are doing. Unless you have some type of physical limitations, your physician will probably give the green light.

Required Walking Equipment and Accessories

In order to enhance your aerobic walking exercises, you will need:

Apparel – Whatever your wear should be comfortable and lightweight. You don't want to wear anything tight where your skin cannot breathe. Clothes that are made from cotton are good to wear.

If you are a night walker, wear light clothing and use reflective tape if you are sharing the road with vehicles. They will be able to see you. Not too many people walk at night, but if you do, have a partner. It's dangerous to walk by yourself when it's dark.

Walking shoes – When you start walking, you want to feel comfortable. Your walking shoes should be lightweight and durable. Get a pair that have a round heel and are breathable. Water resistant shoes are good if you will be walking in various kinds of weather.

Love Your Heart, Love Aerobics

Using a pedometer will help you to measure your walking distance. It's easy to use. You just program it and attach it to your belt or waistband. Once you have finished walking, you will know how long you have walked for that time period.

While you are walking, you should find out what you target heart rate is. It's important to know that so that you can either increase or decrease how fast you are walking. There are several accessories you can use for that purpose:

• Ankle weights

• Hand weights

• Wrist weights

In order to calculate your heart rate, you would take your age and remove that number from 220. Then you would take the difference and multiply it by the percentage you are looking to shoot for.

Increased Aerobic Walking

The more walks you do the fitter you will get. So this means you will have to eventually start walking every day. Make it a habit and gradually work your way up to that point.

Stick with the 150 minutes or so per week. As you continue at that pace, you can work your way up to 45 minutes or an hour per week.

Keep up with your progress. Take daily readings of your aerobic walks. You will see how far you have come since you started. Once you see your numbers looking the same, you will know that it is time to make some adjustments to your fitness routine.

Once you start making strides, reward yourself. Some people go out to eat when they have reached an achievement. Some say you should skip the food. If you're not careful, you can overeat or eat the wrong foods. More rewarding things that you can do is go shopping for yourself, going to a movie, or getting your nails done or a massage. These are things that are worthy of rewards.

3. Bicycling

You can get several benefits from cycling. Not only will you be able to see the sights from the outside and get some fresh air, but you can also get fit. In addition to that, you will burn calories and fat.

Riding a bicycle is a great way to enhance your cardiovascular system. It also allows you not to deal with the pollution coming from other vehicles.

On a bicycle, when you are going uphill and riding at a high intensity, you will be able to gain muscle and burn fat from your body. Your small and large muscles will develop more and get even stronger. When your muscles get more developed, your body will look fit, lean and strong.

This aerobic exercise can also increase your metabolism. You will burn more calories when your metabolism is higher. Even after you have finished for the day, you will still burn more calories.

The core of your body will gain strength, including the muscles in the back and your abdomen. With that, bicycling helps you to have good posture and be able for your body to have a balance.

This is good for activities and tasks that require the weight of your back. Bicycling can help you to increase the capacity of your aerobics, reduce risks of certain illnesses, such as blood pressure, cholesterol and cancer.

Riding a bicycle on a regular basis can help your muscles to get oxygen easier. So when you are doing strenuous tasks or exercises, you won't feel long winded.

There are people who ride bicycles that use them to increase their cardiovascular system. If you are one of those who have a crippling ailment such as arthritis, you may not be able to do activities because of your knees. While toning the leg muscles, bicycling is also used to tone the backside.

There are people who will a stationary bicycle, but that does not help as much as one where you can ride around the park and around town for your fitness workout. When you are using one where you can move around more, you can shift your weight to your legs. You have to be careful that you don't overdo it for fear of damaging your knees.

There is an increase in people that are bicycling in order to stay fit. Because they are concerned about their health and how they look, this aerobic exercise has emerged as one of the more popular activities that people like and want to do. Plus, since you don't use gas, there's no reason why you can get fit and burn calories with a bicycle.

Cycling outdoors is good to do when:

• The weather is presentable

• If you have time to ride your bike

• If you can ride on a cycle path

• If you like to ride outdoors

• If you don't mind the vehicles and possible traffic

You can also go cycling on tracks, forests and beaches. Whatever way that suits you should be ok, as long as you are getting in a fitness workout.

Check Your Bicycle First

• The height of the seat should be comfortable and high enough for you. If it's too low, let it up. If it's too high, let it down.

• Check the handle bars to make sure that they care comfortable enough for you and that you can reach them.

• Your seat should also be comfortable enough for you to sit down.

How to Start Riding Your Bicycle

Just because people own a bicycle does not mean that they know how to get started riding it. It is not difficult to get started on your journey to aerobic fitness.

Start out with short rides. Don't overdo it or overwhelm yourself for trying to break a record by going for longer trips. Starting out, shoot for at least an hour's ride up to 15 miles. Of course, you can do less than that, depending on your strength.

It's easier to start riding your bike in the park. While you're riding, you can go sightseeing at the same time. You will see areas that you had not seen before or just passed by without giving it a second look.

Love Your Heart, Love Aerobics
Once you start, you won't want to stop. This is a great way of getting a workout while being able to see lovely views on the outside.

CHAPTER 10 - HOW TO AVOID INJURIES

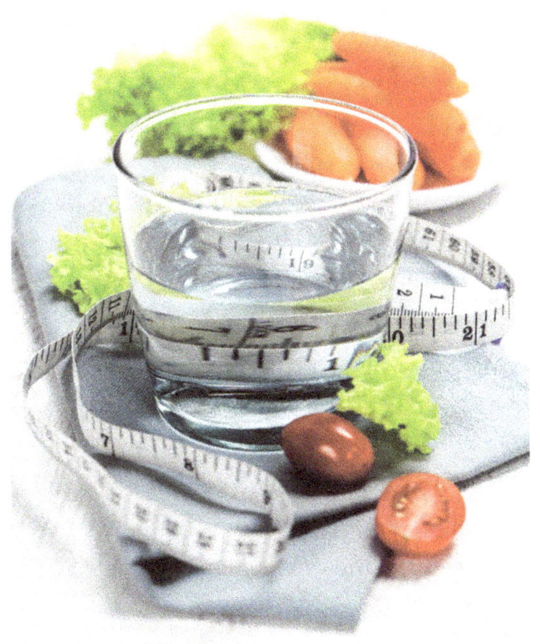

Some people think of cycling as dangerous. That's because some of the bicyclists may not adhere to the road rules and can incur injuries.

One thing that you must do when you are on a bicycle is to wear a helmet. You want your head to be protected in the event of an accident. The brain Is very delicate and once it gets injured, the recovery process could be lengthy.

It is very common to find out that bicycle injuries can affect your knees. The knee injuries can affect anyone that rides a bicycle.

Other bicycle injuries can be caused by:

• Not being prepared to ride for long stretches

- The gear you using is too high for where you are riding

- You are not fitting on bicycle correctly and the saddle is not adjusted for your height

- Trying to ride too many inclines in the beginning stages of riding your bike

Make sure that the height of your saddle on the bicycle is not too high when you are riding. It should be at a height where you are comfortable as you use your pedals. If you are too high on the saddle, you can experience knee pain at the posterior. The height of the saddle should not be too low, either. The knees anterior will be affected.

The saddle should be fitted correctly so that you can sit on it right. If it is not, your muscles could go out of balance. To avoid an injury where you overuse your muscles while riding, set the saddle at an angle between 25 – 35 degrees.

If the ride is uncomfortable for you, then you won't be able to get very far with your aerobic bicycling. You can end up with other "overuse" injuries by overdoing it on the bicycle.

- Chronic nerve damage – riding you bike for long periods of time without resting

- Palm damage, carpal tunnel syndrome – overuse of bike riding

- Bicycle seat neuropathy – numbness, pain in the groin area; can lead to erectile or sexual dysfunction

Cynthia Lopez
Hydration is Key

It's important to stay hydrated while before and during your running exercise. This can prevent you from suffering heat related illnesses. If you don't drink enough, you can get tired, uncoordinated and your muscles can start to cramp. You can also pass out, especially in warm weather.

You can also experience a heatstroke, exhaustion from the heat. When you are running, you need to know how much you are drinking through the entire process.

Prior to you running, you should drink at least 24 ounces of water. This should be done at least an hour before you start. If not water, drink something that does not contain caffeine. Twenty-four ounces of water should be enough to get you started. If you drink too much, this can end your exercise regimen because you will be forced to go to the bathroom.

While you are running, drink at least eight ounces of fluids that don't contain caffeine. This should be done at least every 20 minutes. If you are running for more than an hour and a half, include a sports drink to replenish sodium and minerals.

Have a water bottle or something similar that you can carry your fluids in during your running exercise. This is for those who don't have access to water on their route while they are running.

After you have finished running, you will need to replenish the fluids that you sweated during your exercise. Check the color of your urine afterwards. If the color is dark yellow, drink more fluids. Your urine should be a light yellow.

These tips will help you to stay hydrated and able to run the course. The last thing you need is to pass out while you are out and about.

About the Author

Cynthia Lopez is a gym instructor and weight loss coach. Her clients include personalities, housewives and even teens and children struggling with weight loss.

Cynthia was born in Mexico. After college, she moved to the US to find a job but unfortunately, she couldn't find a decent job that is enough to pay the bills. Good thing she has always had the knack for aerobics and that became her lifesaver.

Today, Cynthia runs her own gym. She also accepts consulting services.